I0775244

INTRODUCTION: EMBRACING THE JOURNEY FROM SKINNY TO SCULPTED

Welcome to "From Skinny to Sculpted: A Macro Counting Journey for Serious Muscle," a comprehensive guide designed to transform your physique and empower you with the knowledge to build serious muscle. This book is not just about gaining muscle; it's about understanding the science behind it, making informed nutritional choices, and embracing a lifestyle that aligns with your bodybuilding goals.

Understanding Your Body's Potential

Every journey starts with understanding where you are and where you want to be. This book is tailored for individuals who might feel they are too skinny or struggle to gain muscle mass. You will learn how to tap into your body's potential for transformation through targeted nutrition and effective training.

The Science of Muscle Building and Nutrition

Muscle building is an art backed by science. It's essential to grasp the biological processes that enable muscle growth, such as protein synthesis, hormonal influences, and the impact of specific nutrients on your body. Understanding these concepts will help you make smarter choices throughout your muscle-building journey.

A Comprehensive How-To Guide

This book is designed to be a step-by-step guide:

Macronutrient Breakdown: You'll get specific numbers and ratios of proteins, carbohydrates, and fats tailored for muscle gain. For instance, a common starting point might be consuming 30% of your calories from protein, 40% from carbohydrates, and 30% from fats. However, we'll dive into how to fine-tune these ratios based on your body type, activity level, and goals.

Product Recommendations: From protein powders to fitness apps, you'll get recommendations on the best products that can support your journey.

We'll cover which supplements are worth considering and how to choose the right ones.

Meal Plans and Recipes: To ease your macro counting journey, the book includes sample meal plans and delicious recipes that align with your macro targets.

Workout Routines: A muscle-building diet works

best when paired with an effective training regimen. We'll provide detailed workout plans that complement your nutritional efforts.

Tracking Progress: Learn how to track your progress, adjust your diet and workouts, and overcome plateaus.

By the end of this book, you'll have a clear understanding of what it takes to transform your body from skinny to sculpted. You'll not only be equipped with theoretical knowledge but also practical tools and strategies to apply in your daily life.

This journey requires commitment, patience, and perseverance. But with the right mindset, tools, and information, achieving your dream physique is within reach. Let's embark on this transformative journey together!

CHAPTER 1: THE BASICS OF MACRONUTRIENTS

Understanding Proteins, Carbohydrates, and Fats

To embark on a successful muscle-building journey, understanding the role of macronutrients – proteins, carbohydrates, and fats – is crucial. Each plays a unique role in muscle development, energy provision, and overall health.

Proteins: The Building Blocks of Muscle

Function: Essential for muscle repair and growth. Proteins are made up of amino acids, which help in the synthesis of new muscle tissue.

Sources: Lean meats, dairy, eggs, legumes, and plant-based alternatives like tofu. Supplements like whey protein can also be beneficial.

Recommended Intake: For muscle building, aim for about 1.6 to 2.2 grams of protein per kilogram of body weight per day.

Carbohydrates: The Primary Energy Source

Function: Carbs are broken down into glucose, providing the energy required for intense workouts.

Sources: Whole grains, fruits, vegetables, and legumes.

Recommended Intake: Approximately 4 to 7 grams per kilogram of body weight, depending on your activity level.

Fats: Essential for Hormonal Balance and Nutrient Absorption

Function: Fats are vital for absorbing fat-soluble vitamins and producing hormones, including testosterone, crucial for muscle growth.

Sources: Avocados, nuts, seeds, fatty fish, and olive oil.

Recommended Intake: About 20% to 35% of your total daily calories should come from healthy fats.

The Role of Each Macronutrient in Muscle Building

Proteins for Muscle Repair and Growth: Post-exercise, your muscles are primed for repair and growth, a process fueled by protein. Consuming adequate protein ensures your body can rebuild the muscle fibers torn during workouts, leading to increased muscle mass.

Carbohydrates for Energy and Recovery: Carbohydrates replenish glycogen stores depleted during workouts. They also play a role in insulin release, which helps transport amino acids into muscle cells, aiding in recovery and growth.

Fats for Hormonal Health and Sustained Energy: Healthy fats are essential for maintaining hormonal balance, which is crucial for muscle growth. They also provide a more sustained energy source, beneficial for endurance and overall health.

In the following sections, we'll delve into how to calculate your specific macro needs based on your body type and goals, and provide tools for tracking your intake effectively. This chapter serves as the foundation upon which your macro counting journey will be built. By understanding and manipulating your macronutrient intake, you can optimize your diet for muscle gain and overall health.

CHAPTER 2: GETTING STARTED WITH MACRO COUNTING

Macro counting is a powerful tool for anyone looking to gain serious muscle. It involves tracking the number of proteins, carbohydrates, and fats you consume each day. This chapter will guide you through calculating your macros and using tools to track them effectively.

How to Calculate Your Macros for Muscle Gain

Calculating your macros is a crucial step in tailoring your diet to your specific muscle-building goals.

Here's a step-by-step process:

Determine Your Caloric Needs: First, calculate your Basal Metabolic Rate (BMR) – the number of calories your body needs at rest. Then, factor in your activity level to get your Total Daily Energy Expenditure (TDEE).

Set Your Macro Targets: For muscle gain, a common macro ratio is 40% carbohydrates, 30% protein, and 30% fats. Adjust these ratios based on your body's response and goals.

Translate Ratios into Grams: Based on your caloric needs and the macro ratios, calculate how many grams of each macronutrient you need. Remember, protein and carbohydrates contain about 4 calories per gram, while fats contain about 9 calories per gram.

For example, for a 2,500 calorie diet with a 40/30/30 split:
Carbohydrates: 40% of 2,500 = 1,000 calories ÷ 4 = 250 grams
Protein: 30% of 2,500 = 750 calories ÷ 4 = 187.5 grams
Fats: 30% of 2,500 = 750 calories ÷ 9 = 83.3 grams

Tools and Apps for Tracking Your Intake

Manually tracking your macros can be challenging. Fortunately, there are tools and apps designed to simplify this process:

MyFitnessPal: Allows you to log your meals and automatically calculates the macros for you. It has a large database of foods, making it easier to find and track what you eat.

Cronometer: Offers detailed nutrition tracking, including micronutrients, which can be particularly useful if you're also concerned about meeting your vitamin and mineral needs.

Fitbit: While known for activity tracking, Fitbit also offers features to log your food and track your macros.

Remember, consistency is key in macro counting. It might seem overwhelming at first, but with practice, it becomes a natural part of your routine.

As we move into the next chapter, we'll explore how to structure your meals throughout the day for optimal muscle gain, including pre and post-workout nutrition.

CHAPTER 3: STRUCTURING YOUR MEALS FOR MUSCLE GAIN

Meal Planning Strategies

To effectively build muscle, it's not just about hitting your daily macro targets; it's also about when and how you consume those macros. This chapter focuses on structuring your meals to optimize muscle growth.

Frequency and Timing: Instead of three large meals, consider eating 5-6 smaller meals spread throughout the day. This approach can help maintain steady energy levels and ensure a continuous supply of nutrients to your muscles.

Balancing Macros: Each meal should include a balance of proteins, carbs, and fats. Proteins are essential for muscle repair, carbs for energy, and fats for hormone production and nutrient absorption.

Pre-Workout Nutrition: About 30 minutes to an hour before

your workout, consume a meal high in carbohydrates and moderate in protein to fuel your session. For example, a banana with a scoop of whey protein can be effective.

Post-Workout Nutrition: Post-workout meals should focus on protein to aid in muscle repair and carbs to replenish glycogen stores. A meal with lean protein (like chicken or fish) and a complex carb (like brown rice or sweet potatoes) is a great choice.

Specific Meal Ideas and Recipes

Here are some meal ideas that align with the muscle-building macro goals:

Breakfast: Omelet with vegetables and a side of whole-grain toast.

Lunch: Grilled chicken breast with quinoa and steamed broccoli.

Dinner: Baked salmon with sweet potato and a green salad.

Snacks: Greek yogurt with berries, nuts, or a protein shake.

Meal Prep Tips

Meal prepping can save time and ensure you stay on track with your nutrition goals:

Plan Ahead: Dedicate a day to prepare and portion out your meals for the week.

Storage: Invest in quality storage containers
to keep your meals fresh.

Simplify: You don't need to cook every meal from scratch.
Simple, whole foods can be just as effective.

Pre and Post-Workout Nutrition

Understanding what to eat before and after workouts is crucial:

Pre-Workout: Aim for a mix of carbs and protein. Avoid high-fat
foods as they can slow digestion and make you feel sluggish.

Post-Workout: Focus on protein for muscle repair
and carbs to replenish energy. Hydration is also
crucial, so drink plenty of water.

By strategically planning your meals and incorporating the right
balance of macronutrients, you can significantly enhance your
muscle-building efforts. Remember, nutrition is just as important
as your workout regimen in your journey from skinny to sculpted.

In the next chapter, we'll delve into the specific types of exercises
and training routines that will complement your nutritional
efforts and help you achieve your muscle-building goals.

CHAPTER 4: EFFECTIVE TRAINING FOR MUSCLE DEVELOPMENT

Weight Training Fundamentals

Building muscle requires more than just lifting weights; it requires a strategic approach to strength training. This chapter will cover the essentials of effective weight training for muscle gain.

Progressive Overload: The key to muscle growth is progressively increasing the demand on your muscles. This can be achieved by increasing the weight, altering the number of repetitions or sets, or changing the exercise complexity.

Compound Exercises: Focus on compound movements like squats, deadlifts, bench presses, and pull-ups. These exercises work multiple muscle groups simultaneously, offering more efficient muscle-building potential.

Consistency and Routine: Establish a regular workout schedule. A common approach is a split routine, where you target different muscle groups on different days (e.g., 'leg day,' 'chest day').

Form and Technique: Proper form is crucial not only for muscle development but also for injury prevention. Consider working with a trainer to learn the correct technique.

Creating a Workout Plan that Complements Your Diet

Your workout plan should align with your nutritional strategy:

Pre-Workout Meals: Ensure your pre-workout meal or snack fuels your upcoming physical exertion.

Intensity and Duration: Tailor your workouts' intensity and duration to match your energy levels, which are influenced by your diet.

Rest Days and Nutrition: On rest days, focus on slightly reducing calorie intake, particularly carbohydrates, as your body won't require as much energy.

Sample Workout Routines

Here's a sample beginner workout routine:

Day 1: Chest and Triceps

Bench Press: 3 sets of 8-10 reps

Dumbbell Flyes: 3 sets of 10-12 reps

Tricep Dips: 3 sets of 10-15 reps

Day 2: Back and Biceps
Pull-Ups: 3 sets of 6-8 reps
Bent Over Rows: 3 sets of 8-10 reps
Bicep Curls: 3 sets of 10-12 reps

Day 3: Legs and Shoulders
Squats: 3 sets of 8-10 reps
Lunges: 3 sets of 10 reps per leg
Shoulder Press: 3 sets of 8-10 reps

Remember, these are just guidelines. Modify the routine based on your fitness level and goals.

Tracking Progress and Adjusting Your Routine

Monitor Your Strength Gains: Keep a workout log to track increases in weights and reps.

Listen to Your Body: Pay attention to how your body responds and adjust your routine accordingly.

Periodization: Consider varying your training intensity and volume over time to avoid plateaus and overtraining.

In combination with your macro counting and nutritional strategies, this workout approach can significantly aid your journey from skinny to sculpted. The right balance of nutrition and exercise will unlock your body's full muscle-building potential.

In the next chapter, we'll explore how to overcome plateaus and make adjustments to your nutrition and training over time.

CHAPTER 5: OVERCOMING PLATEAUS AND COMMON CHALLENGES

Gaining muscle is a journey marked by progress and occasional stagnation, commonly known as plateaus. Understanding how to navigate these plateaus and other challenges is crucial for continuous growth and development.

Adjusting Macros and Workouts Over Time

As your body changes, so too do its nutritional and exercise needs. Here's how you can adapt:

Reassess Your Macros: As you gain muscle, your body's caloric needs will increase. Regularly recalculating your macros can ensure you're consuming enough to support further growth.

Change Your Workout Routine: Your muscles adapt to stress over time, reducing the effectiveness of a consistent routine. Introducing new exercises, altering your sets and reps, or changing your workout split can provide new stimuli for growth.

Dealing with Stalls in Progress

When progress stalls, it's essential to analyze both your diet and your training regimen:

Nutritional Audit: Ensure you're not only hitting your macro targets but also getting a wide range of micronutrients. Sometimes, small deficiencies can impact overall performance and recovery.

Intensify Your Workouts: Incorporate techniques like supersets, drop sets, or pyramid sets to increase intensity.

Rest and Recovery: Overtraining can lead to plateaus. Ensure you're getting enough rest and not pushing your body beyond its recovery capacity.

Managing Expectations

Building muscle is a gradual process:

Realistic Goals: Set achievable goals to keep motivated. Remember, significant muscle gain takes time.

Patience and Persistence: Stay committed to your

routine, even when progress seems slow.

The Role of Rest Days

Rest days are just as important as workout days:

Muscle Repair and Growth: Muscles grow during rest, not during workouts.

Active Recovery: Engage in light activities like walking or yoga to promote blood flow and aid recovery.

Psychological Aspects of Muscle Building

The mental aspect of bodybuilding is often underestimated:

Mind-Muscle Connection: Being mentally present during workouts can enhance muscle activation.

Dealing with Frustration: Find ways to manage frustration and keep a positive mindset.

In conclusion, overcoming plateaus and challenges in muscle building involves a mix of strategic adjustments, mental resilience, and an understanding of your body's needs. Being adaptable, patient, and committed is key to pushing beyond these hurdles and continuing your journey from skinny to sculpted.

In the next chapter, we'll dive into the importance of rest and recovery, and why they're crucial components of your muscle-building journey.

CHAPTER 6: THE IMPORTANCE OF REST AND RECOVERY

Building muscle isn't just about what happens in the gym or at the dining table; it's equally about what happens during periods of rest. In this chapter, we delve into the critical role of rest and recovery in the muscle-building process, covering everything from sleep to active recovery methods.

The Role of Sleep in Muscle Growth

Sleep is paramount for muscle recovery and growth.

During deep sleep, your body releases growth hormones that are essential for muscle repair and building.

Sleep Duration: Aim for 7-9 hours of quality sleep per night. Consistency in your sleep schedule is also crucial.

Sleep Environment: Create a sleep-conducive environment - dark, quiet, and cool. Consider investing in a comfortable mattress and pillows.

Pre-Sleep Routine: Establish a relaxing pre-sleep routine to signal your body that it's time to wind down. Avoid screens, caffeine, and heavy meals close to bedtime.

Active Recovery and Muscle Repair

Active recovery refers to engaging in low-intensity exercise during rest days. It helps in muscle repair by increasing blood flow, which aids in nutrient delivery and waste removal from muscles.

Activities for Active Recovery: Include walking, light cycling, yoga, or swimming in your active recovery days.

Stretching and Mobility Work: Incorporating stretching or yoga can improve flexibility, reduce soreness, and enhance your range of motion, contributing to better performance in strength training.

Hydration: Staying well-hydrated is crucial for recovery. Water helps transport nutrients to your muscles and removes waste products.

Nutritional Strategies for Recovery

Nutrition plays a vital role in muscle repair and recovery.

Protein: Ensure you're consuming enough protein, especially after workouts, to provide the necessary amino acids for muscle repair.

Carbohydrates: Don't shy away from carbs; they replenish glycogen stores, vital for recovery.

Micronutrients: Vitamins and minerals like Vitamin D, calcium, iron, and zinc are essential for muscle health and recovery.

Timing of Meals: Eating a meal rich in protein and carbs after your workout can aid in quicker recovery.

Managing Rest Days

Rest days are an integral part of your training regime.

Scheduling Rest Days: Plan your workout routine to include rest days, allowing different muscle groups to recover.

Listening to Your Body: Pay attention to signs of overtraining like excessive fatigue, decreased performance, insomnia, and irritability. Take extra rest if needed.

Mental Recovery: Use rest days to mentally recharge as well. Meditation or engaging in hobbies can be excellent ways to reduce stress.

The Mental Aspect of Recovery

Stress Management: High levels of stress can impede recovery. Techniques like deep breathing, meditation, or even leisure activities can help manage stress levels.

Positive Mindset: Maintain a positive attitude towards your body's need for rest. Embrace rest days as part of your progress.

In summary, rest and recovery are as crucial as the workouts themselves in your muscle-building journey. They allow your body to heal, muscles to grow, and energy levels to replenish. By prioritizing adequate rest, engaging in active recovery, and following nutritional strategies that support muscle repair, you lay the groundwork for continuous growth and avoid the pitfalls of overtraining.

In the next chapter, we'll explore the various supplements available to support muscle growth, how to use them safely, and determine which ones are worth incorporating into your regimen.

CHAPTER 7: SUPPLEMENTS TO SUPPORT MUSCLE GROWTH

In the realm of muscle building, supplements can be a valuable addition to your diet and workout regimen. They can help fill nutritional gaps, enhance performance, and speed up recovery. However, it's important to approach supplementation with knowledge and caution.

Identifying Beneficial Supplements

The supplement market is vast, but not all supplements are necessary or effective. Here's a guide to some of the most beneficial supplements for muscle growth:

Protein Supplements: Whey, casein, and plant-based proteins can help you meet your daily protein requirements, especially post-workout.

Creatine: One of the most researched supplements, creatine can enhance muscle mass, strength, and exercise performance.

Branched-Chain Amino Acids (BCAAs): BCAAs are critical for muscle growth and recovery, especially if you're exercising in a fasted state.

Omega-3 Fatty Acids: Found in fish oil supplements, omega-3s can aid in muscle recovery and joint health.

Vitamin D and Calcium: Important for bone health and muscle function, especially if your diet is lacking in these nutrients.

Beta-Alanine: This amino acid can improve exercise performance and reduce muscle fatigue.

Navigating the World of Supplements Safely

While supplements can be beneficial, it's essential to use them wisely:

Quality Over Quantity: Choose high-quality products from reputable brands. Research their reviews and certifications.

Dosage and Timing: Follow the recommended dosages and consider the timing of intake for optimal benefits (e.g., taking protein post-workout).

Consult a Professional: Before starting any supplement, especially if you have underlying health conditions or are taking medication, consult with a healthcare professional.

Natural Nutrition First: Aim to get most of your nutrients from whole foods. Supplements should complement, not replace, a balanced diet.

Debunking Supplement Myths

The supplement industry is rife with myths and exaggerated claims. It's important to approach supplements with a critical mind and understand that they are not magic pills for instant muscle growth. Real gains come from consistent training, proper nutrition, and adequate rest.

Supplements and Individual Needs

Everyone's body responds differently to supplements. What works for one person might not work for another. Pay attention to how your body responds and adjust accordingly.

In conclusion, supplements can be a helpful addition to your muscle-building arsenal, but they should be used thoughtfully and as part of a well-rounded approach to diet and exercise. Remember, there are no shortcuts to building muscle – supplements are just one piece of the puzzle.

Next, we'll move on to long-term strategies for sustained muscle growth, ensuring you're equipped for the ongoing journey in muscle development.

CHAPTER 8: LONG-TERM STRATEGIES FOR SUSTAINED MUSCLE GROWTH

Building muscle is not just a short-term endeavor; it requires a long-term commitment and a strategy that evolves as you progress. This chapter focuses on advanced approaches to ensure continuous growth and avoid stagnation.

Beyond the Basics: Advanced Macro Adjustments

As your body changes, so too should your nutritional strategy. Advanced macro adjustments involve fine-tuning your diet based on your evolving goals and physiological responses.

Periodic Recalculation: Regularly reevaluate your caloric needs and macro ratios as your body weight and composition change.

Carb Cycling: This involves alternating between high-carb days (typically on training days) and low-carb days (on rest days) to maximize muscle growth while minimizing fat gain.

Targeted Supplementation: Depending on your progress, you might need to adjust your supplements. For instance, increasing creatine intake during intense training phases or adding glutamine for recovery.

Lifelong Fitness: Balancing Diet, Exercise, and Lifestyle

For sustainable muscle growth, it's crucial to balance all aspects of your health and lifestyle.

Holistic Approach: Beyond diet and exercise, ensure you're managing stress, getting adequate sleep, and addressing any other health issues that could impact your muscle-building journey.

Regular Health Check-ups: Keep tabs on your overall health with regular medical checkups, especially if you're consuming supplements or making significant dietary changes.

Adapting Workouts: Continually challenge your muscles by changing your workout routines. Incorporate different exercise modalities like resistance training, HIIT, or even sports.

Beyond Muscle: Understanding Body Composition

As you advance in your journey, focus on body

composition rather than just muscle mass.

Body Fat Percentage: Consider tracking your body fat percentage to get a clearer picture of your fitness progress.

Functional Fitness: Incorporate exercises that improve not just strength but also balance, agility, and flexibility.

Setting New Goals and Evaluating Progress

As you achieve your initial goals, set new ones to stay motivated. This might mean increasing muscle mass, improving muscle definition, or achieving specific strength targets.

Performance Metrics: Keep track of your lifting progress, endurance levels, and other performance metrics.

Regular Photo Documentation: Take regular photos to visually track your progress.

Coping with Plateaus and Staying Motivated

Even the most experienced bodybuilders face plateaus.

Mixing Things Up: Sometimes, all you need is to change your routine or try a new approach to nutrition.

Seeking Inspiration: Stay inspired by following bodybuilding communities, reading about fitness, or working with a coach.

In conclusion, sustained muscle growth is a journey of continuous learning and adaptation. It's about fine-tuning your approach as you go along and maintaining a balance between all aspects of your health and fitness. As you grow in your bodybuilding journey, remember that change is the only constant, and adaptation is the key to progress.

In the next chapter, we'll explore real-life success stories to inspire and guide your journey from skinny to sculpted.

CHAPTER 9: SUCCESS STORIES AND INSPIRATIONAL JOURNEYS

Real-Life Transformations

This chapter is dedicated to real stories of individuals who embarked on their journeys from skinny to sculpted, offering insights and inspiration. These narratives highlight the challenges, strategies, and triumphs encountered along the way, providing a realistic perspective on what it takes to achieve significant muscle gains.

Diverse Backgrounds: The individuals featured come from various backgrounds, ages, and lifestyles, demonstrating that muscle-building success is achievable for a wide range of people.

Strategies and Techniques: Each story includes specific strategies and techniques that were pivotal in achieving their goals, such as particular diet plans, workout routines, and mental resilience tactics.

Before and After: Accompanied by before-and-after photos, these stories visually depict the transformations, offering a powerful testament to the effectiveness of disciplined training and nutrition.

Learning from Others' Experiences

The success stories serve not just as motivation but also as practical guides. They offer valuable lessons:

Common Challenges: Understanding the challenges others faced can prepare you for similar obstacles, such as plateaus, motivational dips, and balancing fitness with other life commitments.

Adaptation and Change: Many stories show how individuals had to adapt their approach over time, reinforcing the need for flexibility and learning in your muscle-building journey.

Holistic Approaches: These narratives often highlight the importance of a holistic approach, including mental health, recovery, and the role of a supportive community.

How to Apply These Lessons

As you read through these stories, consider how the lessons can be applied to your own journey. Identify strategies that resonate with you and think about how you can incorporate them into your routine.

Setting Realistic Goals: Inspired by these stories, set goals that are challenging yet achievable. Use the SMART (Specific, Measurable, Achievable, Relevant, Time-bound) framework to define them.

Staying Inspired: Keep these stories as a source of motivation. When you feel like skipping a workout or straying from your diet plan, remind yourself of what others have achieved and what you're capable of.

Sharing Your Journey: Consider documenting and sharing your journey. Not only can this hold you accountable, but your story could also inspire others in the future.

In conclusion, these success stories are a testament to the transformative power of disciplined muscle-building efforts. They serve as a reminder that while the journey from skinny to sculpted requires dedication and hard work, it is undoubtedly achievable and profoundly rewarding.

In the next chapter, we will prepare you for what comes after achieving your initial muscle-building goals, setting the stage for ongoing fitness and body sculpting.

CHAPTER 10: PREPARING FOR WHAT COMES NEXT

After achieving significant progress in your journey from skinny to sculpted, you may wonder, "What's next?" This chapter focuses on setting new goals, transitioning to maintenance or further development, and ensuring your achievements are sustainable over the long term.

Setting New Goals

Re-Evaluate and Reflect: Take time to assess the progress you've made and what you've learned about your body and preferences.

New Objectives: Depending on your experience, you might set goals for further muscle gain, fat loss, or enhancing specific aspects of your physique.

Functional and Athletic Goals: Consider setting goals beyond aesthetics, like improving strength, endurance, or flexibility.

Transitioning to Maintenance or Further Development

Maintenance Phase: Learn how to adjust your diet and training to maintain your new physique. This might involve slightly lowering your calorie intake or altering your workout intensity.

Continuous Development: If you decide to continue building muscle, consider advanced training techniques like periodization or undulating training patterns for continued progress.

Staying Injury-Free: Incorporate strategies to protect your body from injuries as you push into more advanced training realms.

Lifelong Fitness and Health

Balanced Lifestyle: Ensure that fitness remains a part of your lifestyle without overshadowing other aspects like social interactions, hobbies, and relaxation.

Nutritional Balance: Find a diet that you can adhere to long-term, one that balances your fitness goals with enjoyment and health.

Mental Health: Pay attention to your mental well-being, recognizing the importance of self-esteem, body image, and overall happiness.

The Importance of Adaptability

Evolving Strategies: Be open to changing your fitness strategies as your life circumstances, goals, or body responses change.

Continuous Learning: Stay informed about new research and developments in fitness and nutrition.

Sharing Your Knowledge and Experience

Inspiring Others: Consider sharing your journey to inspire and help others. This could be through social media, blogging, or even coaching.

Community Involvement: Engage with fitness communities as a source of support and a way to offer guidance to those starting their journeys.

Preparing for the Road Ahead

Remember, fitness is a lifelong journey. It's not just about reaching a specific goal but about adopting a sustainable, healthy lifestyle. As you transition from achieving your initial muscle-building goals to setting new ones, keep in mind the principles of balance, health, and continual growth.

In conclusion, "From Skinny to Sculpted" is more than a physical transformation; it's about embracing a lifestyle that celebrates strength, health, and continual self-improvement. Your journey doesn't end here; it evolves into something even more rewarding.

CONCLUSION: EMBRACING THE LIFELONG JOURNEY OF FITNESS AND GROWTH

As we wrap up "From Skinny to Sculpted: A Macro Counting Journey for Serious Muscle," it's important to reflect on the journey you've embarked upon. This path is not merely about physical transformation; it's a journey of discipline, self-discovery, and personal growth.

More Than Just Muscle

While the primary goal of this book was to guide you from a skinny physique to a sculpted one, the journey encompasses more than just muscle gain. It's about adopting a lifestyle that prioritizes health, wellness, and balance. The lessons learned here extend beyond the gym and the kitchen; they're about cultivating a mindset geared towards lifelong improvement.

The Role of Consistency and Adaptation

Consistency is Key: Your results are a direct reflection of your consistent efforts in nutrition, training, and recovery.

Adaptation is Necessary: As your body changes, so too should your approach. Be willing to adapt your training, nutrition, and recovery methods.

The Ongoing Nature of Fitness

Fitness is not a destination but a continuous journey. As you reach each goal, new ones will emerge. Your relationship with your body and your understanding of fitness will evolve, and with it, your methods and practices.

A Lifelong Commitment to Health

Remember, the ultimate goal is a sustainable, healthy lifestyle. This journey is about finding a balance that works for you—one that allows you to enjoy life while being the best version of yourself.

Sharing Your Journey

Consider sharing your experiences and knowledge gained. Whether it's through social media, in your local gym, or with friends and family, your journey could inspire and motivate others to embark on their own fitness paths.

Gratitude and Reflection

Lastly, take a moment to appreciate the work you've put in. Reflect on where you started and where you are now. Celebrate your achievements, learn from the challenges, and look forward to the road ahead with excitement and determination.

As you close this book, remember that your journey from skinny to sculpted is unique to you. It's not just about the physical transformation; it's about building strength, resilience, and confidence that transcends the gym. Carry these lessons forward, and embrace the lifelong journey of fitness and growth.

Thank you for choosing "From Skinny to Sculpted" as your guide on this transformative journey. May your path forward be rewarding and fulfilling in every aspect.